To Pa—

What Is Beautiful:

Secrets from a Personal Shopper

Blessings to you,
Jica

What Is Beautiful:
Secrets from a Personal Shopper

by

TICA TALLENT

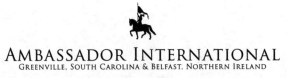

AMBASSADOR INTERNATIONAL
GREENVILLE, SOUTH CAROLINA & BELFAST, NORTHERN IRELAND

www.ambassador-international.com

What Is Beautiful
Secrets from a Personal Shopper

© 2011 by Tica Tallent

Printed in the United States of America

ISBN: 9781935507765

Cover Design by David Siglin of A&E Media
Page Layout by Kelley Moore of Points & Picas

Scripture taken from the NEW AMERICAN STANDARD BIBLE®, Copyright © 1960,1962,1963,1968,1971,1972,1973,1975,1977,1995 by The Lockman Foundation. Used by permission.

AMBASSADOR INTERNATIONAL
Emerald House
427 Wade Hampton Blvd.
Greenville, SC 29609, USA
www.ambassador-international.com

AMBASSADOR BOOKS
The Mount
2 Woodstock Link
Belfast, BT6 8DD, Northern Ireland, UK
www.ambassador-international.com

The colophon is a trademark of Ambassador

Endorsements

Tica Tallent is a style and fashion educator who has taught hundreds of clients to define and develop their own personal style. She is a captivating speaker with an effective approach to style that transcends all shapes, sizes and lifestyles. Her seminars have shown us how to avoid costly wardrobe mistakes and to create a wardrobe to love!

~Haley Sitton, Director of AnMed Health Foundation
Research and Donor Development

Tica has been a personal friend of mind for twenty five years. Her physical beauty is obvious, but her spirit is even greater. She has lived each of her experiences to serve as a vehicle of Jesus' love.

~Charlotte Sams, Personal lifelong friend

"Style is a novelty perceived by others." Tica's extraordinary eye for detail and quality has been enhancing individual personal style for over a decade. She is truly a novelty maker of personal Beauty and Style!

~Melisa Morris Glenn, President and Owner,
The Feathered Nest Linen and Interior Design
Comfort Keepers Franchise Owner

Tica Tallent is a fashion expert—however, her most important quality is a genuine caring and service approach towards each individual she interacts with—Tica truly knows how to give the gift of service to others.

~Janet Cantrell, HR/Operations Manager,
Belk

I LOVE this lady!!! I think Coco Chanel must have been speaking about Tica Tallent when she said a girl must be two things...classy and fabulous. This woman covers both of those easily. There have been several queens, duchesses, and princesses of note in recent years but I can assure you there is only ONE Tica Tallent! She is gracious and sweet as southern iced tea but known as a mover and shaker! All you need is to spend a few minutes with Tica and not only will her character and integrity shine out, her ability to inspire and make things happen will amaze you. In a nutshell, this lady is INCREDIBLE! Her actions always cause people to dream more, learn more, do more, and become more. Simply put, SHE IS FABULOUS and I'm blessed to know this lady!

~Jonathan Dickson, Actor, New York, N.Y.

Contents

Preface

THIS BOOK IS A SUMMARY of the knowledge I have gained as a personal shopper for fifteen years at a major department store. It is also a summary of the hundreds of professional wardrobe presentations given to civic organizations, church groups, college faculties and students, sororities, debutantes, moms of preschoolers, secretaries, auxiliaries, and societies of every kind! As a public school teacher with a Master of Education, a professional model and modeling class instructor, a wife, mother, and an observer of humanity for sixty-five years, I have also added my personal tips for living a successful and blessed life.

I hope the information I share with you on self-evaluation, including body type, hair, and makeup, your basic style, critiquing your wardrobe, cleaning out your closet, selecting lingerie, finding your best colors, using accessories, and making your best impression will help you in your quest to become your most beautiful *you*. I even include my own twenty-five tips for shopping for success. Consider this book your "personal shopper in your pocket"!

I have learned beauty is an asset, just as intelligence, wealth, charm, and athletic ability are assets. It can be used to attract attention, it can be used to get your foot in the door, but it *cannot* assure one of good self-esteem or success in life. I have seen many beautiful people with tattered, unhappy lives. Good self-esteem comes from knowing that *each* of us is a *unique creation*. God has planned our genetics exactly as they are. It is our responsibility to use each of our assets to serve others. As you learn to present your best self through the tips in this book, always let the love of God shine through you to others, and your *true* beauty will never fade.

Acknowledgments

IT IS WITH A HEART full of love and true gratefulness that I thank Andrea (my agent and beautiful daughter), Scott (my son and sun), and Larry (my cherished husband) for their encouragement as we have fulfilled my true dream of sharing my knowledge of fashion, while most importantly sharing my love of God.

I thank Ambassador International for having faith in me and taking a chance on an unknown writer.

I appreciate so much the constant support from my dear family and friends, without whom I would have many times given up on this venture!

And I thank *you*, the reader. I hope you will be informed and entertained, but more importantly I pray you will be *blessed*.

Introduction

"For I am confident of this very thing, that He who began a good work in you will perfect it until the day of Christ Jesus" (Philippians 1:6).

THANK YOU FOR PICKING UP this book. With all the self-help information in stores and on the Internet, I am honored you chose this one! I feel this book will make your life easier, teach you a great deal about the woman you are now, and truly make your life more beautiful.

At sixty-five years old, I have had many people ask me, "How do you look so young?" As a personal shopper for a major department store for fifteen years and a professional model for twenty years, I have shared the information that follows through modeling classes and state and national professional dress seminars. I am excited about sharing these secrets with you.

We are going to examine your hair and makeup, critique your wardrobe, identify your best colors, determine your body type, discuss your personal style, take a walk through the lingerie department, learn how to use accessories to your advantage, and build a wardrobe that works for your life now. I even have a shopping list for you to use and tips for making a great first impression. Consider this book your portable personal shopper.

You don't have to be born with perfect features to live your best life. But how you present yourself to the world says a lot about not only how you view your world but also how you view yourself.

As we begin our journey together, here are a few basic questions for you to consider:

1. Can you go into a large department store and select the one item or items that you need to complete your wardrobe?

2. Are you drawn immediately to age-appropriate, figure-flattering clothing?

3. When you look in your closet each morning, can you quickly put together an amazing ensemble perfect for the day's activities?

4. Do you have special events—interviews, weddings, reunions, or first dates—coming up and you know exactly what is appropriate?

5. Is your wardrobe truly current with who you are right now—as you are reading this? (Find a mirror quickly!)

6. Are you confident using accessories to your advantage: jewelry, scarves, handbags, and shoes?

7. Do you still get approving looks and smiles from men and women?

8. (For those over 55) Are most people astonished when you ask for your senior discount?

If you answered "no" to any of the first seven above, this book is for you. During fifteen years as a personal shopper I have helped hundreds of women and men find their best look. And I have found that many tricks of the trade are *not* public knowledge. So let us begin! You may want to go ahead and prepare your modest acceptance speech for when the compliments keep coming your way.

Notes

"What is beautiful is good, and who is good will soon be beautiful."

—Sappho

"Taking joy in living is a woman's best cosmetic."

—Rosalind Russell

CHAPTER ONE

Evaluating Your Hair and Makeup

"For by Him all things were created, both in the heavens and on earth, visible and invisible . . . all things have been created through Him and for Him" (Colossians 1:16).

WHETHER YOU ARE A VERY young woman in your 20s, or in your 30s, 40s, 50s, or 60s—or older—we all have one thing in common. We all want to be respected as human beings of worth, and we desire to project that image of confidence, whether working from home as a business owner or parent, working at a job in our community, volun-

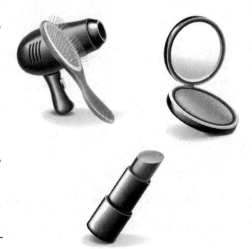

teering our time, or enjoying retirement. As we move through these stages of life, we do not lose ourselves—we simply improve ourselves.

As you begin this self-evaluation, I am asking you to find a full-length mirror and look at yourself for the first time. Don't look immediately at the flaws you wish you could change (and even swimsuit models have them, trust me!). You may have some things you wish you could change; but rather than focus on those areas, take what God has given you and make the most of it. Stand straight and tall, if you can, and focus on your hair and face. As you look at only your hair and face, ask yourself the following:

Hair

1. Is your haircut/color flattering and easy to style?

2. Can you change your style quickly with a headband, rubber band, barrettes, or hat if needed?

3. Have you had your face shape analyzed to know which hair length is best for you?

4. Do you have a professional that can cut your hair with precision?

5. Do you often use a back mirror to look at your hair from every angle?

6. Do you own hair products (only 2–3) that enable you to change your look?

I will admit I am not a hair person. I have a dear friend who changes her hair every year or two and can do more with three inches of hair than I can with a full mane! For those of you in my friend's category, this information might be redundant, but for the rest of us that are challenged, it may be helpful.

I have learned through the years that our hair does change along with the rest of our bodies. The thick, easy-to-manage hair you had in your twenties may be a thing of the past. This certainly doesn't mean that those of us fortunate enough to have hair cannot work with it successfully. And after speaking to many, many women, I know that our hair professional is right up there with our dearest family doctor. Moving to a new state without her hairdresser is major stress for any woman!

In spite of changes in your hair quality, one of the most important people you can have in your life is your hairstylist—or as older ladies used to say, your beautician. I have learned that you can find your special person (if you don't already have this person) with research. Keep your eyes open as you go through your day, looking for the one lady that has the style and/or color you admire and think you can copy. Go right up to her and ask her for the name and phone number of her hairstylist. I have done this often and the woman always responds with a big smile and helpful advice. (What lady would *not* find this a compliment?) When you make your appointment, be as helpful as you can to express your needs to your stylist. Bring pictures from magazines if you have them. But be realistic. I had to learn sadly years ago that I would never look like Farrah Fawcett no matter how my hair was cut!

As you look for a new style, consider your particular natural hair: curly, straight, prone to frizz, etc. Also, consider your face shape: oval, round, oblong, heart-shaped, and square are a few basic shapes. If you do not know your face shape, a quick trick is to look in your bathroom mirror and trace your face on the mirror with soap (or anything that will wash off easily). You will be able to see your face shape easily. When you have your next appointment with your stylist, tell him or her about your basic face shape and how much time you have to work with your hair. If you are a busy mother or a professional woman with many responsibilities, you may not have much time to spend.

Also, consider the weather where you live. When we lived in Houston for four years while my husband was in school, I wore a wig every Friday! The tremendous humidity there made it very difficult to control my naturally wavy hair. Many salons provide software you can use to actually see yourself in different haircuts and colors. So if you have been wondering what it would be like to be a blonde or a redhead, try this software first. You will save money and your hair!

You can also go to a wig boutique and have fun trying on wigs and making mental notes about color and cut. I once followed this advice and tried on an auburn wig since my two children have beautiful auburn hair. One of the young ladies in the room said I looked exactly like Carol Burnett! That was quite a compliment! (However, I did not look like myself, so I stuck with the hair color I have, with highlights.) I also know several ladies who have invested in hair pieces or wigs for those days they just need some extra help.

At your hair appointment, notice the shampoo and hair products your stylist uses. Many times he or she will be glad to give you samples before you buy—but do not be a product junkie, as I was for years, thinking my great style would come out of a bottle. Your professional stylist has been trained for years to do what he does, so ask questions at your appointment and even make notes, if necessary.

This might be the time to invest in professional hair equipment as well as bottled products. Owning a professional hair dryer, curling iron, and other tools will at least give you a more equal playing field!

Also, keeping your equipment clean, including your brushes and combs, is imperative. Change the filter on your hair dryer and wipe your curling iron with a warm, damp cloth (make sure both are unplugged first!). Wash your brushes and combs in a sink filled with shampoo and warm water; rinse well after washing and air-dry.

Remember this last thought concerning your hair and your stylist: I have learned that the most expensive stylist is *not* always the best one for you. You can find someone you can afford that can do a fabulous job. Just remember: you are the buyer, and you may shop around until you find a perfect match. When you do find that perfect person (until you or the stylist moves) remember to give him or her a great tip and verbal thanks when you are pleased. You might even find out the stylist's birthday and bring a small gift—and of course, during holidays it's imperative to remember your special person with kindness. Let your stylist know his or her importance in your quality of life!

At this point I want to mention your manicure and pedicure. These are as important as your hairstyle as you put together your best self. If you are fortunate to have a great manicurist, as I have had for twenty years, please value this person. If you cannot afford this service right now, you can certainly take care of your own nails—but just do it! Nothing damages an overall appearance more than unkempt nails or nail polish chipping off. (Thank you, Sherry!)

Face/Makeup

1. When you look at your face, can you tell you have emphasized your best features?

2. If you wear makeup base, is it a perfect match and consistency for you?

3. Is your skin care regimen a must, morning and night, and perfect for your skin?

4. Do you have a good dermatologist?

5. Do you always wear sunscreen when exposed to the sun?

6. Does anyone ever compliment you on your skin—or just your makeup?

7. During the last ten years, have you made necessary changes in products or regimens that suit your skin now?

I have learned as a makeup artist while teaching modeling classes that healthy skin is beautiful skin. A lifestyle that includes lots of water, plenty of exercise, and low stress levels is important to healthy skin and a healthy life.

Moisturizer and sunscreen are your skin's best friends. The expert at the makeup counter or at your private makeup store can help you select the best moisturizer for you. Actually, too much moisture cream is not good for your skin, as it can clog your pores or cause your skin to sag prematurely. Deciding if you are oily or dry or a combination of both is a job for the experts—with your feedback, of course.

The goal of makeup application is to cover imperfections simply and quickly and to add interest to your best features. Your personal style, whether classic, sporty, romantic, dramatic, or fashionista, certainly affects your choices. Your makeup for a tennis match and your makeup for a debutante dinner would certainly be different, but you should be able to apply makeup for both with ease. Again, the experts at the makeup counters in most department stores or makeup boutiques will help you at no cost. So use these resources and make sure what you are currently using is best for you. As we age, it's true that our needs change, and we can see this truth at the makeup counter as well. If you develop a friendship with a makeup artist, she can also give you a heads-up on upcoming gifts with purchase and many times drop special surprises in your bag!

Realize also that every free gift or seasonal color may not be for you. If you are a warm season and this year mauve and hot pink are big trends, just wear what you have for now. As with everything else, the tide will eventually change and your colors will be popular again. This principle holds true with the "cool woman" who is facing brown and nude lip colors and blushes.

Here's a final note concerning makeup application: keep all of your makeup brushes, sponges, and puffs spotlessly clean. If they are washable, wash with your face cleanser. If not, replace when soiled. Your face will thank you. During the day, try not to touch your face unless applying makeup. You will prevent breakouts and even illnesses by breaking this habit. And it is true that you must thoroughly cleanse your face twice a day, morning and night. Never, ever sleep in your makeup. This will clog pores—and you might even lose precious eyelashes by ignoring old mascara.

Notes

"Do you know the difference between a beautiful woman and a charming one? A beauty is a woman you notice, a charmer is one who notices you."

—Adlai E. Stevenson

"You can take no credit for beauty at sixteen. But if you are beautiful at sixty, it will be your soul's own doing."

—Marie Stopes

CHAPTER TWO

Critiquing Your Wardrobe

"Therefore, take up the full armor of God, so that you will be able
to resist in the evil day. . . ." (Ephesians 6:13).

MOST WOMEN THAT I HAVE met through my job as a personal shopper or
the ones I have met during wardrobe seminars have one thing in common:
they have closets filled with items
they do not wear—either they don't
fit their body now or they don't fit
their lifestyle. Actually, if you are
truly honest, you probably wear one
tenth of what you are looking at as
you review your closet.

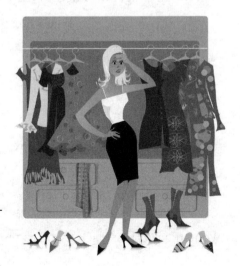

As a personal shopper, I was
asked on occasion to come to customers' homes and clean out their
closets. I normally did not do this,

but on the few occasions that I did for special friends or family, the above held true. So many ladies hold on to items because of special memories. Yes, some of us are very sentimental! But even if you wore that special dress to your daughter's wedding ten years ago, if it doesn't fit you now and you know you won't be wearing it again, take heart—you have pictures. Let it go!

Now I realize we do need special clothing for special events: formal cocktail affairs, sports events, or just working out in the yard. But your closet should be arranged in a way that you can see quickly where things are when you need them. Anything that is uncomfortable, not flattering, outdated, or worn-out should be removed. If you are on a diet and want to be a size six—but aren't—slide those size sixes under the bed, but *don't* hang them in your closet. Also, don't save clothing for years and years thinking the style will come back. It may, but your figure probably won't be the same (sorry).

I've heard it said, "If you remember wearing a trend the first time, don't wear it again." There is truth in that adage!

So, as you look closely at your body *now*, make sure your clothing

1. Fits

2. Is well-liked

3. Is your color

4. Works for your lifestyle now

5. Is in good repair

As women, we tend to over-buy our favorite items. For instance, no woman needs five black T-shirts, ten pairs of jeans, or four pairs of brown boots. This is where a personal shopper is needed. And I am right here to help you!

Let's begin. Go to your closet on your day off (or for one hour, if that's all you have) and get started. Take everything—and I mean everything—out. Lay all the items in your closet from top to bottom out of your traffic area until you can get to each one. After vacuuming and dusting your closet, strip down to your underwear and start trying on each one. Hang back only the items in your closet that pass the five criteria mentioned earlier. The items that do not pass will form piles: one pile for selling or donating, one pile for mending or altering, one pile for saving (the size sixes!), and, alas, one pile for throwing away. (No one wants your old yard shoes that are falling apart).

As you hang your passable items back in your closet, remember to put the items closest to you that you wear most and your formal outfits in the back. Of course, this placement depends on how your racks are arranged, but I'm thinking ideal scenario here! If you work outside your home, your work clothing should be together, blazers together, blouses together, and so on. It will help you if you also hang them by color. That way you won't be in a hurry and show up in navy pants and a black blazer! You can hang pants and skirts on stackable hangers to save room. All dresses should be together. If you have a dress with an accompanying jacket, don't hang them together. Hang your dress with the dresses and the jacket with the jackets. That way you will be forced to mix and match. And it goes without saying that your gym clothes should be together.

There is an exception to this rule of arranging clothes. Once after working as a personal shopper for five years, I had an older lady call to ask me to come to her home to help her clean out her closet. I did tell her

I had to charge for my services, but she was grateful I would come. Her husband had died the year before and she had retired from her banking job. When I arrived at her home, I saw two closets (her husband's and hers) filled with her work suits. I asked her to empty them all out and then we started trying on. I placed her jackets and tops in one closet and her skirts and other bottoms in the adjoining closet. I was pleased with our job when we had finished. However, when I saw her later in the month she said, "Tica, I cannot find what goes with what in my closet. I am totally confused." So I'm mentioning this to those of you that do not like to mix and match as I do. The closet police will not come and chastise you! You are arranging items for *your* ease, not mine.

I find that putting my shoes in clear plastic boxes works well. Boots also should be visible. If you have room, hang your scarves on a scarf hanger (or pant hanger) within sight. Jewelry can be displayed as you can in your environment: in a drawer, on a jewelry hanger, in a box, in plastic bags, or arranged on velvet compartments inside a covered space. However, review it often. It will help if you have all of your silver together, gold together, and pearl pieces together.

When you purchase a new piece of jewelry, think of your basic, favorite colors of clothing. At the home jewelry show of a good friend, I recently bought a bracelet that had five different colored strands of my favorite colors. I've worn it often since!

When you have tried on everything in your closet and organized what you have, you will be amazed. This is what you are really wearing anyway! All the other items are just taking up space. At this point you may have a "need" list. If this is your year to purchase a new coat or suit, when you go shopping it will be a planned purchase—and you will be using your money wisely. Remember to count the number of times you will be wearing a piece of clothing as you consider its price. (In the business we call that cost per wear.) But before you hit the mall in earnest, let's talk a bit about color.

Notes

"Magenta.

Within the family of red.

It's who I am.

From the flame of my hair

To the passion in my soul

Running through my veins

To the tips of my toes.

Alive."

—Andrea Tallent

"Beauty without virtue is a flower without perfume."

—French Proverb

CHAPTER THREE

Gaining Color Clarity

"Then Jesus again spoke to them, saying, 'I am the Light of the world; he who follows Me will not walk in the darkness, but will have the Light of life'" (John 8:12).

As I mentioned earlier, color is paramount. You need to know above all if you are warm or cool and be able to list quickly five of your favorite colors. No amount of money spent on a wardrobe will be worthwhile if you do not know what colors look great on you. And this knowledge is *not* known by everyone. I have seen people in the public media wearing the wrong colors and have shouted to myself, "Where is their stylist?!"

Before we start, let me add a disclaimer: If you are very young or very beautiful and/or very good at adapting your makeup to go with a certain color, you probably can wear any color you like. I've never met a ten-year-old child that had trouble with color! And it is true that *most* of us *can* wear any color in the spectrum—it is the intensity of the color that separates us.

To be succinct, you are either warm or cool. Warm colors have a yellow undertone, cool colors have a blue undertone. An easy way to think of this is to imagine pouring a little yellow or blue paint into a basic color and watch the change! A basic green (in a pack of eight crayons) could turn yellow green (warm) or blue green (cool).

I have worked with light brunettes that could wear warm and cool colors equally, but that was not the usual case. When a new customer called me for an appointment, I always asked them if there were colors they loved or did not wear. If they truly didn't know, when they arrived at their appointment we would go out on the sales floor and I would drape warm and cool colors on them. You can do this for yourself. Sample warm test colors could be olive or yellow green, camel, ivory, peach, and shades of gold, yellow, and orange. Sample cool test colors could include blue-green, pink (including hot pink and rose), pure white, purple (including lavender), dark blue/red, dark gray, and burgundy.

Please notice that I did not mention black. I am a firm believer that most women can wear black. However, I have dressed some very, very pale ladies that could not—and also as we age we must remember that even though we need to contrast our lighter hair color, some older ladies find black too harsh for their lighter complexions. Let your experienced eye be the judge here. And you can soften a look that is not quite right with a beautiful scarf or necklace (more on that later). Also, use your eye color as a tool to point you in the right direction. The right color will truly make your eyes pop. Think of the compliments you receive when you wear certain colors—and if someone asks you if you are ill and you are not, that is *not* your color!

There are some colors that do indeed look good on everyone, such as watermelon, aqua, true blues, and usually black. This principle is good to know when selecting an outfit for groups such as bridesmaids, choirs, dance or sports groups, etc.

Once you know your best colors, shopping (and packing) is so easy. You can purchase a necklace or scarf with confidence, knowing it will blend with everything you have. And as you pack for that special trip, choose neutral solids in your colors and you will have lots to wear. Our men have known this for years!

As you understand your coloring and your best colors, you will understand why you have such good luck at certain boutiques. I would bet that their buyer also is your coloring! If you are a warm lady and are browsing through aisles of dark blues and reds, stark zebra prints, and hot pinks, you may need to change stores or at least departments. Buyers, of course, need to know this so they can appeal to everyone and increase their sales. Also, shopping with a family member, friend, or husband that is not your coloring is a challenge. They will consistently show you items in the colors that look fabulous on *them*. That is why I recommend shopping alone when you are truly on a mission!

And what should we do with the "perfectly good" slacks or skirts that are not in our color palette? Well, dear, go ahead and wear them! Just be sure to add tops (blouses, jackets, sweaters, or T-shirts) that are complementary near your face. Or you might even organize a clothing swap with friends! Two of my dear friends and I did this at Christmas this year instead of purchasing new items for each other. We looked in our closets and found things that we did not use that we thought they would love. Not only did we save money, the gifts were special because they were things really from us, not the store window!

The Power of Color

A science has surely been made on the impact of color in room decor, doctors' offices, and even work environments. But color also plays an important part in making your first impression! When meeting some-one for the first time in a business setting, think darker, solid colors. Of course your clothing personality, body type, and skin tone affect the color choice, but in an interview situation, always think calm, conservative team player, and you are on your way!

Black

What it does: Demands respect and makes you feel more in control.

How it works: Referees wear black to show they are in charge. You can give off that same vibe when you're taking your driving test or on a job interview.

Blue

What it does: Helps relieve stress and improves your ability to communicate.

How it works: Blue will calm you down when work or friends and family are driving you crazy! Navy blue is a true American classic.

Red

What it does: Can make you feel assured and courageous.

How it works: The Chicago Bulls would probably be a decent team no matter what color their uniforms were, but wearing red gives them a psychological edge over their opponents.

Green

What it does: Helps you see the bright side and improves your self-image.

How it works: If you're down in the dumps, sleep on green sheets!

Yellow

What it does: Can boost your brain power and help you focus.

How it works: Yellow helps you block out distractions and focus on the task at hand. You can feel the color's energy just by sitting on a piece of yellow poster board while you are reading!

To aid in color selection, a sampling of color squares has been included at end of the book.

Notes

*"The future belongs to those who believe
in the beauty of their dreams."*

—Eleanor Roosevelt

*"Beauty is not in the face; beauty
is a light in the heart."*

—Kahlil Gibran

CHAPTER FOUR

Identifying Your Body Type

"The eye is the lamp of your body; when your eye is clear, your whole body also is full of light. . . ." (Luke 11:34).

NOW THAT WE HAVE ASSESSED our needs for our face and hair and discovered our best colors, it is nice to look again at that full-length mirror and really notice what we are trying to dress! When we were teenagers, many of us selected swimsuits by color; but, alas, time does change things. But the advantage we have now is we have learned tricks to turn back the clock, or at least fool most of the people most of the time!

When I worked as a professional shopper, body type was my most important clue as to how to begin my job. When a client called for the first time, I would always ask them their height, approximate size, and if they ever wore a petite. After asking color information, that alone would give me a start.

Forgive me if these are basics you already know, but I have certainly found *not* everyone knows the following. Most ladies fall into general

categories: Regular Ladies, Petite Ladies, or Today's Woman sizes. However—and this is a big *however*—when you go to a department store, keep
an open mind. Body type is much more important than age. I have fitted ladies in their sixties in the Junior department because of their height
and body type. I have also fitted some pre-puberty boys with girls' shoes
because they were more narrow. My point is, knowing your body type
will free your mind to look at the options available for you. In fact, many
ladies are two departments. They can be petite on the top and regular
or women's sizes on the bottom or vice versa. Most women that I have
helped didn't know this. And did you know that most stores are very un-
derstanding when you find a petite blouse and ask to carry it to another
department to find slacks or a skirt?

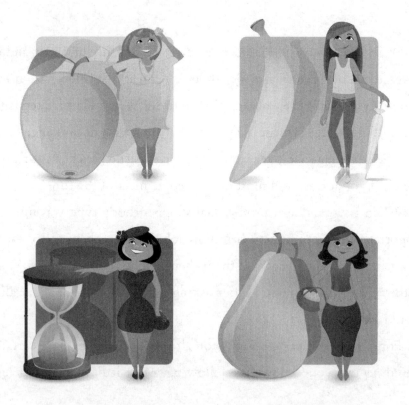

A sweet lady came to my office a number of years ago after her phone interview—with her three skinny sisters. This lady had told me over the phone she was a size 18 because that was the department where her sisters had taken her to shop. Since that was the largest size she saw, she ended up buying muumuus that draped over her body, literally hiding herself in fabric. After sending her sisters away, I started trying to fit her in slacks. We started with her 18 R (regular) then went to the Today's Woman department where everything was too long. And voila—I handed her a Woman's Petite (that she had never heard of in her life) and although it was tight, we continued to 20 and then 22. I just wish you had been there with me when this dear little lady tried on pants that were the right length and actually had a belt that she could buckle! She literally went wild! She spent $1,000 in about two hours that day on a bright yellow suit (her color) and lots of pieces that mixed and matched and that *fit*. When her sisters came back, they were totally in awe. The back trouble that she had complained about only a couple hours before was gone. She was strutting outside my office doing quarter turns for all to see! That is retail therapy at its best! Before she left I showed her where to find her size in the store. I will admit I haven't seen her again, but if she is reading this book, I want her to know that she was an encouragement to many women.

So, let's not underestimate body type! Even if you are a young woman, most of us are not a perfect size. If you happen to be a perfect size, you are probably not reading this book—and if you are, you can skip this chapter and give the book later to one of your friends (if you have any!).

I have already mentioned the different departments and sizes available for you and the need to keep an open mind to everything that might fit. Mothers, that includes you trying to fit your preteens. I did fit an eight-year-old, chubby little girl in T-shirts from Petite ladies once. So, hopefully this information will be valuable to you as you shop for family members as well!

When making a selection on a possible item, after trying it on, *always* look at yourself in a back mirror. If the store does not provide one, bring your own. Even a compact will do. Many outfits may look good from the front but might bulge or be unattractive from the back. I am telling you now what your best friend might not tell you! Also, sit in your new outfit, even if it is a dress. There will be a chair or stool somewhere in the building. Your tops and bottoms should fit smoothly, even while sitting. And ladies that are going for job interviews, this tip is even more essential for you. When you sit in front of a full-length mirror, you will see what your interviewer is seeing! Just ask yourself if this is the image you are trying to project.

So what is the perfect length for your dresses, skirts, and jackets? Ah, that depends on you—not the latest magazine! In modeling class as a young woman, I was taught to stand in front of a full-length mirror with bare legs and a large piece of poster board to cover most of them. Place the poster board at your ankles and slowly raise it, showing your legs at each angle. (It may help if you have on the shoes you normally wear.) Your eye is good enough to know when to stop and where the curve of your leg is most attractive. Personally, I have long, slim legs. In middle school I was told they were "skinny" and was always afraid to show them off. When I became an adult I learned they were an asset—but I also learned that Bermuda shorts with a wide leg opening were not for me. I could wear short shorts—at the beach of course—or capris.

You too must learn which items are best for your body. Some stereotypes are just not true. Large women can wear flowers, petites can wear palazzo pants. It all depends on the length and width of what you are dressing. Be careful when using a double-breasted jacket if you are endowed in that area.

Where your jacket stops on your hip is important, especially if you are using more than one color. And now we are back to colors! This is especially relevant when considering body type. Your eye looks in the direction of lines and colors. That's why low V-neck tops are sexy. The eye goes straight to cleavage! Horizontal lines or patterns will cause your eye to go back and forth and also add width to that area. If your bust and hips are a similar size, you will have a slightly easier time than the girls that have a big discrepancy. Also, if you have a naturally small waist, you must have the latest and prettiest belts available!

Keep in mind also as you assess your body that you may be short-waisted or long-waisted. This simply refers to the length between your belly button and your shoulders. A long-waisted person has more body than usual to cover from her waist up. A short-waisted person has less body than usual to cover from her waist up. You can find this out by standing sideways in a full-length mirror and wrapping an oblong scarf around your middle. Use a back mirror if necessary. Placing the middle of the scarf in the center of your back, bring the two ends forward. If your belly button is below where the two ends join, then you are long-waisted. If your belly button is above where the two ends join, you are short-waisted. If the two ends join at your

belly button, you have an average waistline. This is important information to know when selecting clothing colors and especially belts.
Belts that are the same color as your top or bottom will add width
to that area. For example, a short-waisted woman wearing a white
blouse and black skirt would want to select a white belt to help visu-
ally lengthen her torso; a long-waisted woman would select a black
belt to help shorten her torso.

And what should you do if you think you are truly "unfittable"?
(And yes, I have had customers that really were.) This is when alterations are truly needed. If you are in a wheelchair or have other
special needs or if the Lord just got creative with your shape, and if
you do not have a seamstress, you do need to find one! The ladies at
the department store where I worked for so long were truly magi-
cians. And a snip here or there can make a mediocre outfit fabulous.
Once I was looking for a formal dress for myself and found one in
my favorite color on the clearance rack. After trying it on I saw the
problem. It had a small "cut-out" right in the center of the breast
area. Now, I don't know where you live, but in my small town if
you are my age and wear a dress with a cut-out between the breasts,
you *will* be talked about. I took this dress to my friend in alterations
and she very simply (in two minutes) sewed up the hole. The design
was not disfigured in the least, and I got the dress for twenty dollars
and felt very pretty the night I wore it! (And if you can sew *yourself*,
good for you!)

So, do not dismay if you are short-waisted or long-waisted or have
unusually short or long legs or arms. We are all fabulous creations. It is
just a little harder for some of us to figure this out! And, as a side note,

before you go to alterations, you should consider laundering first if the item is washable. I bought a warm-up suit not long ago that was a little large for me. The washing directions said wash in cold water and dry on low. I washed in warm water and dried on low. It fits perfectly now! (I was lucky!) But, seriously, before you have pants hemmed, etc., wash them first if you can and try to stick with the directions. It may save you an alteration. This is true when an item is a little small and the fabric is stretchable. While it is wet, lay it flat and just tug a little where you need a little more room and let it air-dry. I have been lucky more often than not with these endeavors.

Notes

*"He has made everything beautiful in its time.
He has set eternity in the hearts of men."*

—Ecclesiastes 3:11

"To me, fair friend, you never can be old,

For as you were when first your eye I eyed,

Such seems your beauty still."

—William Shakespeare

CHAPTER FIVE

Defining Your Basic Style

"O Lord, You have searched me and known me" (Psalm 139:1).

WE ALLUDED TO YOUR CLOTHING personality earlier when we discussed makeup. At this point in our journey we are going to identify in more depth your basic style. You can be classic, sporty, romantic, dramatic, or fashionista, to mention just five personal styles. I'm sure there can be as many styles as the next generation can imagine! But for now put yourself into one or a combination of the above. It is helpful to know what general style you are as you enter a shopping mall and also great information for someone else as they shop for you. Has anyone ever come back from a shopping trip and told you, "I saw something that looked *just like you!*" If so, that is great—there is a *you!*

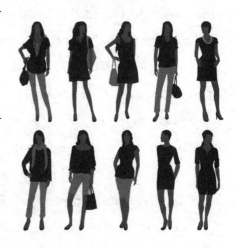

If you are a classic lady, regardless of fashion trends that come and go, you will be comfortable in suits, dresses, tops, and bottoms that are not overly frilly. Many of your clothes will be solid colors, with many neutral colors. The classic lady definitely is not boring. Quite the opposite is true. This is the woman you think of often when you think of great style. She, in fact, could be a designer herself! Often her accessories make a statement and she does not over-do them. A great necklace (including pearls of course), a wonderful scarf, or a leather belt might be her signature. She is fortunate because her clothing will last for a long time (if her figure does also).Certain designers are meant for the classic lady and she knows how to find them. She would prefer to have one new fabulous item than a new wardrobe any day.

The sporty woman does not, indeed, have to be athletic. Her style is simply casual. She feels best with the wind in her hair! This doesn't mean she doesn't hold an important job or can't live in a big city. But this woman is most comfortable when *she* is comfortable. She usually doesn't wear suits, and if she does, her choice of top underneath might be an oxford shirt or a T-shirt with a scarf. She loves cotton, corduroy, and tweed. Her accessories can be cutting-edge though, and you might find this lady wearing a hat for fun or layers of costume necklaces. When trends come out in force, she is willing to try them out regardless of her age. When the sporty woman is happy, she is many times the life of the party. Choosing clothing for her is very easy, if you do know her colors!

The romantic female knows she is a female! She loves silky fabrics, lace, and velvet and—depending on body type—is drawn toward ruffles. She tends to have more dresses and skirts than pants and spends a great deal of time when selecting these items. You would never see the romantic woman in flannel pajamas, even in winter. This woman likes to wear her clothing snugly. She is the woman that often loves to be a little late and make an entrance. She is totally comfortable in her own skin and doesn't mind showing some of it (in good taste). As a personal shopper for fifteen years, I have concluded that there is a little "romantic female" in most women!

And, yes, the dramatic woman is definitely exciting. Her clothing can be any of the above but usually is an unexpected combination. She uses contrast well, knowing her body type, and understands how to make a statement with her brightest colors. This woman many times can find items and put them together and make them work, while the rest of us just could not. She is the lady with the tattoo or multiple earrings. You might find her in patterns that don't match or polka dots and prints to-gether. But the dramatic woman has learned from much experimenting (usually as a teenager) how to use shock appeal in good taste. Even if her cleavage is showing, women still love her! You probably won't find flat shoes in this lady's closet, unless she just can't walk in any others. She might even find her accessories at the local farmer's market—but on her, they will be *fabulous*!

And last, but certainly not least, is the fashionista. Many times this is a younger woman, but it doesn't have to be. It is simply the woman who truly loves the newest in fashion. This lady will wear trends a year before they hit the stores, simply from instinct. She, more than any of the others listed, is not defined by her colors. She may fly to New York or L.A. just to shop. Whatever is "in," she has it and knows how to work it! As a personal shopper, I did not fit this woman often because she didn't need me! She is the most difficult to buy for because her taste is way ahead of her peers. This woman is always very bright and articulate and a true trendsetter in her own right. Excitement truly surrounds her and she usually has a big following of friends that long to copy her!

I hope you could find at least a snippet of yourself in the descriptions above. All of this I learned early on while fitting ladies as a personal shopper. When my customer made her purchases and left my office, I always made notes for myself as to her preferences. When she returned at her next appointment, I was fortified with her exact style and saved us both lots of time.

When you are wearing clothing that flatters your body type, your coloring, and your natural style, you will truly feel more comfortable and confident. Our goal with clothing in general is for you to look great, not just your clothing. If someone immediately notices what you are wearing without noticing your beautiful eyes or dazzling smile, you might *not* be wearing items that truly complement you. I always tell customers to look in the mirror after trying on an outfit and then close their eyes. When they open their eyes, they should be drawn to their face, not their clothing. You should try this too!

Notes

Notes

"I gave my beauty and my youth to men. I am going to give my wisdom and experience to animals."

—Brigitte Bardot

"She said she usually cried at least once each day not because she was sad, but because the world was so beautiful and life was so short."

—Brian Andreas

CHAPTER SIX

Discovering the Magic of Lingerie

"Beyond all these things put on love, which is the perfect bond of unity" (Colossians 3:14).

NOW, YOU MAY WONDER WHY I am spending a chapter on lingerie. It is because it is so important for your overall look. Lingerie is more than the sexy ad you see in the newspaper. It is more than being attractive to your husband or impressing your friends. Lingerie is the foundation for how our clothing looks on us. I am speaking of lingerie for real life, not for "costumes." Panties, bras, slips, and hosiery will be the basics for planning your fabulous outfit. You can have the perfect sweater dress and great boots to go with it, but if you do not have the correct under-

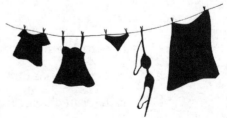

garments, your outfit will not impress; in fact, you might find yourself in *Glamour* magazine with a big X!

First of all, let me begin with this old-fashioned idea: *Your undergarments should not show.* Sorry, Madonna look-alikes! In the lingerie department, you will see signs that say, "To Be Seen." This is for lacy camisoles that really might work under a jacket for evening. But everything else is in the "Private" category. And even though this topic is private, it is truly as important as your outerwear.

BRAS—Most ladies do not wear the correct size. This is what our lingerie professionals tell us. I even went on a "door to door" trip with a bra fitter to some local assisted living communities. As a personal shopper, this was very interesting. I surely did not realize how much a great bra can do for a lady! First of all, most ladies do not realize that the size they wore in college is probably *not* the size they need now. As with all other parts of our body, breasts change. I heard a national talk show speaker say recently that when she got up in the morning and started to dress, she commanded, "Up, girls!" Most of you know what I'm speaking about here! But what most ladies don't know is there is help out there. Whatever problem you have breast-wise, there is a bra for you. This was not my specialty as a personal shopper; I truly sent my customers to the experts in that department. But I have learned personally that if there is a clingy garment you "cannot" wear, it could very well be because of your undergarments!

There are bras for increasing and decreasing your natural endowment. There are even bras to hide the "bulge" in your back. There are convertible bras that can change from strapless to one shoulder, etc. And if you don't mind the discomfort, there are bras to put you in that perfect "10" category. But as for me, I settle for a good, substantial bra that gives me a smooth appearance and doesn't limit my choices of clothing. End of subject.

PANTIES—Some prefer extra support, some waist huggers, some bikinis, some thongs. But as a personal shopper, allow me to just encourage you to not shout to the world your choice in panties! They should work as a smoother under the most clingy outfits. And if you want to be considered for more than "artwork," they should be invisible. Can you bend down to pick up something, ladies, and not show your thongs? God made us to be beautiful to our husbands. But to show the world our choice in panties is too much information—and more than that, it diminishes our worth as women. To be taken seriously in this competitive job market, we do not need to be men, but we need to be women that are taken seriously. If someone in your office is ogling you, that is degrading and disrespectful. Promotions go to the people that can promote the business with no distractions. How can we be respected as equals to men in the workforce if we are always seen as "the lady in thongs"?

SLIPS—Slips are almost gone now. However, if you choose to wear a slip, *use your back mirror*! Let me give a brief illustration. My husband and I were invited to a very formal evening wedding in Charleston, South Carolina, a few years ago. A member of the bride's family arrived in a black limousine. She looked absolutely beautiful—until she gracefully stepped out of the car and her white slip was sticking boldly out of her dark dress! This lady had obviously spent a great deal of time planning her outfit, but a slip ruined what a famous designer had in mind. My point is, ladies, if you decide your skirt is very sheer and unlined and truly needs a slip, make sure it does not show. Once I literally had a slip altered to match the slit in my dress. And it goes without saying that dark clothes need a dark slip, etc. Ah, the importance of that back mirror!

HOSIERY—With a little spray, clothing does not stick, and most items are lined. With self-tanner, our legs can be tan and attractive without hosiery. And here the naturally brown-skinned ladies have a great advantage! Tights and leggings are the popular items to help with leg coverings. So, how do we show our legs to our best advantage without the hose that our mothers and grandmothers depended upon? If you are wearing a skirt or dress and basic shoes, some hosiery is advised for a work environment. In fact, some conservative dress codes insist upon hosiery.

Tights or patterned hosiery is still "cool" and does help for those of us that were not born with beautiful brown skin! Since legs are more than one third of our body, we do need to spend time considering this as we plan our outfits. Know your body type and comfort level as you choose hose, tights, or leggings. (They also come in petite and larger sizes.) And ask your young sales associate or daughters for their advice. Young people love to give advice, and even if it is hard to do, sometimes we need to listen to them! This choice may truly make—or break—your overall appearance!

Also, having a friend who works in the Lingerie department helps immensely. She is a professional that will help you with your correct size and needs and will let you know about upcoming sales. Put this person at the top of your list.

Notes

Notes

*"You don't love a woman because she is beautiful,
but she is beautiful because you love her."*

—Anonymous

"Never lose an opportunity of seeing anything that is beautiful; for beauty is God's handwriting—a wayside sacrament. Welcome it in every fair face, in every fair sky, in every fair flower, and thank God for it as a cup of blessing."

—Ralph Waldo Emerson

CHAPTER SEVEN

Using Accessories

"Your cheeks are lovely with ornaments, your neck with strings
of beads" (Song of Solomon 1:10).

IT STANDS TO REASON IF you picked up this book - and are this far along
in it - you like accessories! But "like" can cover an enormous amount of
ground, as I learned in the trenches fitting ladies day after day. Some felt
totally comfortable adding their own items, and some ladies really were
at a loss and asked me to accompany them to the hat, shoe, belt, handbag, jewelry, and scarf departments. I must admit here that accessories are
my favorite items when it comes to
dressing myself or anyone else. At this
point in our shopping adventures, my
creative juices really started to flow.
(And spending other people's money
was a lot of fun too!)

Accessories are your signature
and many times what others remember about your outfit. I've heard an

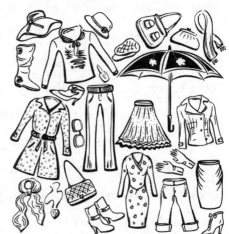

older member of my own family comment on how well-dressed so-and-so was because of her fabulous pin! And as with our other choices of clothing, we need to remember our body type, coloring, and natural style when it comes to choosing accessories. This is also important when we select our eyeglasses. But regardless of your coloring, age, or body type, some ladies just love to dabble in accessories! They have a drawer or hangers full of scarves, lots of real and costume jewelry, fabulous hand-bags, several pairs of designer eyeglasses and/or sunglasses, and the newest looks in shoes and boots. But not all of us have the money or time to fit into the above category. Now is the time for your personal shopper!

As you clean out your closet, your accessories can be sorted through as well. Anything you do not wear should be given to someone that truly might enjoy them. I gave a box of headbands recently to a charity for children. Jewelry is best handed down in your family if possible, and shoes and handbags that you are not using can be sold or donated. I have even given belts to a lady who helped me select wallpaper in my kitchen! So the saying is true: if you don't use it, lose it!

Just as with your other clothing items, you can plan your accessory choices. If you cannot afford a new wardrobe right now, here is the place you can change your look with minimum expense. And this is also the place to utilize those magazines and update your knowledge of what is popular and current. A fabulous scarf or necklace can take ten years off your appearance! People will be looking at that and not your double chin. (Sorry, young ladies who don't get this now—someday you will!)

As for hats, wear them for warmth only or wear them for fun. That choice is totally up to you. But we all have to wear shoes, unless we are fortunate enough to live on an island, and then there are still some rocks!

And as we get older, it is disappointing that we no longer can wear the backless stilettos we used to love. It is true that an outfit just loses some pizzazz when you wear low-heeled shoes even though flats are supposedly the "in" item. But when pain is involved, and some of you are nodding now, we have to make practical choices. You can do as my daughter has taught me: wear your flats in the car until you get to your event and then slip on your fabulous shoes! But at some point in our life our fabulous shoes will be "old lady shoes." The good news is there are many of us now, and the manufacturers are making them prettier and prettier. So, my shoe advice is simple: don't hurt yourself for fashion's sake. You want to take good care of your feet so that they will take care of you for a long time to come. Also, choose real leather whenever you can afford to do so. Your shoes really will last longer and be much more comfortable. This is one place you do not want to cut corners.

A lady's handbag is a very personal item. And those of you that have tried to purchase one for a lady friend understand that fact! I learned in helping women select handbags that most of them like the size they are currently wearing. Also, if you select a handbag the same color as your hair or choose one in one of your basic, neutral colors, it will go with everything in your wardrobe. This is good advice for the lady that doesn't have the time, money, or inclination to change handbags with every outfit. I want to stress here that your shoes and your handbag will do more to add to or subtract from your outfit than any other accessory. If you put on cheap, uncared-for shoes or carry a cheap, plastic handbag, your outfit automatically drops in value even if it is couture! If you choose pleather (not real leather) in your handbags (and I admit, I do have a couple), let them be your fun ones—bright colors, etc.—not your interview or business bag. The same advice is true with leather belts. There is no substitute for real leather if you can afford it!

Jewelry is so personal that I hesitate to even mention it here but it is so necessary that I must! Again, some ladies will not go out for their morning walk without their earrings, and others choose not to wear them at all. But as with other accessories, check the trends but do look closely in your mirror. Your jewelry should not be an undesired distraction in a business setting but a definite addition to an evening dress. Every woman, in my opinion, needs a great pair of silver earrings, gold earrings, and pearl earrings. The length depends on your personality more than anything else. I knew a fabulous lady in her eighties that loved to wear bright, dangling jewelry. And I say, "Go for it, girl!" Your comfort level and clothing personality will guide you here. But when selecting colored pieces, always remember your favorite colors. I love to purchase earrings as a souvenir when traveling. They remind me of my fun trip and are useful when I get home. Since I know my favorite colors (as do you!), I'm sure they will match something I have. And try to match your silver, gold, or pearl earrings with your buttons or belt buckle and you will be totally put together!

My last advice on accessories—and I warned you that I loved them— concerns scarves. Scarves are so misunderstood! Anyone can wear a scarf. There's nothing to it! Now, I understand there are tricky ways of tying them that not everyone knows, but just put one on and let it drape around you. If it is silk, or silky, just tie a simple bow. I wore a silk scarf to a bridge party one time and several ladies asked me how I tied it. Actually, it was just a simple bow that I had twisted to one side. Trends come and go, but scarves will always be with us. If you don't feel comfortable wearing them, maybe you haven't tried the right length or fabric for you. Don't give up on this accessory. Once you start wearing them, you will have bunches—and not be able to part with any of them!

Notes

"A man should hear a little music, read a little poetry, and see a fine picture every day of his life, in order that worldly cares may not obliterate the sense of the beautiful which God has implanted in the human soul."

—Johann Wolfgang von Goethe

"Think beautiful thoughts, and become who you are."

—Scott Tallent

CHAPTER EIGHT

Stealing Savvy Secrets from a Shopping Pro!

"And my God will supply all your needs according to His riches in glory in Christ Jesus" (Philippians 4:19).

ALL RIGHT, WE HAVE EXAMINED our face and hair, checked our body type, and cleaned out our closet! You are on the way to building a great wardrobe.

Now what you need to do is look at what is to come in the next year. This may be hard for some of you, but if so, look at last year's calendar for a better idea. What kinds of events are you expected to attend? Do you have reunions, weddings, showers, special parties coming up? Do you have something appropri-

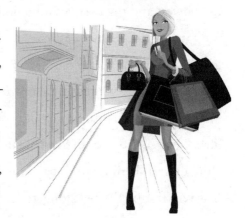

ate for a funeral or last-minute date with a new friend? If you do not, may I encourage you to plan for these events now? When coupons are in the paper or a favorite item is on sale, that is the time to stock up. If you plan ahead for events, you will not be like so many I have helped at the last minute that really couldn't find the "perfect" outfit and had to settle for the best we could find (and often paid too much). Check out sales and new items periodically at your favorite store. You can even ask a sales associate to keep something in mind. But don't count on that being your best resource, as sales associates mean well but are very busy. Be diligent and have your mental list ready so when you find the perfect dress it will be a planned purchase. I used to advise my customers, when they did shop early, not to remove tags and to tape the sales receipt on the original bag that they received. Then if they happened to find something they liked better, they would have everything they needed for an exchange or return.

This does not mean you can *never* vary from your list. And this is where the educated woman wins the "advertiser's dream" contest! Advertisers are paid the big bucks to appeal to your impulse buy. We all know the newest and the best (and the not on sale) items will greet you as you walk in any store. And we are tempted—especially you new mothers and grandmothers out there—to stray from our list. But let me emphasize, as a woman that was truly there from 9:00–5:00: the enjoyment of this item will not equal the stress of going over your budget. So, have your little "mad money" stash for that fabulous blazer or cute new toy for your child or grandchild, but don't come home and lose sleep over something that will not be the best long-term use of your money.

I have made a list that will help you as you try to actually live what you've now learned. Please follow all of the twenty-five suggestions below and you will have a successful shopping experience. All steps on this list are what I actually do when shopping for myself. Good luck!

Tica's List for Shopping with Success

1. Decide where you are going.

2. Have a good idea of how much you plan to spend.

3. Remember to bring your list.

4. *Never* shop with children.

5. Wear something easy to remove.

6. Wear or carry the shoes required. (This especially helps with alterations.)

7. Always wear your best underwear!

8. Take your time.

9. Go alone (or if with a friend, split up).

10. Browse as long as you like.

11. Remember: size is just a number.

12. Keep in mind that many items on sales racks could be sized incorrectly.

13. *Always* drape yourself with the color before trying.

14. Select items to try that aren't your normal choice.

15. Don't buy anything without examining how it is made.

16. Don't buy anything without examining yourself in a three-way mirror.

17. Be able to sit comfortably in your new outfit.

18. Consider "cost per wear" as you assess price.

19. Keep your wardrobe at home in mind.

20. Don't buy an item you already have two of at home! (Of course, *shoes* are the exception!)

21. Spend more money on solid, neutral pieces that you can wear in at least three seasons.

22. Have fun with accessories.

23. Keep receipts.

24. Don't cut tags off until you are ready to wear the item.

25. If shopping for someone else, always ask for a gift receipt.

Notes

Notes

"The longer I live, the more beautiful life becomes."

—Frank Lloyd Wright

"For attractive lips, speak words of kindness.
For lovely eyes, seek out the good in people.
For a slim figure, share your food with the hungry.
For beautiful hair, let a child run his fingers
through it once a day.
For poise, walk with the knowledge
that you never walk alone."

—Sam Levenson

CHAPTER NINE

Making the Best Impression

"Let your light shine before men in such a way that they may see your good works, and glorify your Father who is in heaven" (Matthew 5:16).

GUESS WHAT? YOU ARE ALREADY making an impression! Whether it is a good one or not, I don't know since I don't know you. But I do have a short, true story I would like to share.

Several years ago I received an invitation in the mail for a medical school graduation. The problem was I did not know who this person was! I tried to play detective as you would. I asked my children, my husband (and asked him to ask his associates), our HR person, my friends, and actually everyone I knew at the time *who* this young man was! Not one person knew

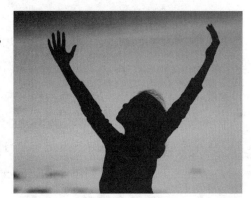

him. Well, since graduating from medical school is quite an accomplishment, whether I knew him or not, I sent him a gift to the address on the invitation.

Two weeks passed and I received a thank-you note (that I still have, by the way). It read, "Thank you so much, Mrs. Tallent, for the generous gift for my graduation. *I will never forget my first grade teacher!*" When I saw his signature—with his nickname—of course I remembered him. It was his official three-part name I didn't remember. But his dear smile and sweet spirit came back in full force when I saw the name I knew.

Well, you can imagine my reaction. And I tell you this story to impress upon you that you will never know, this side of heaven, what kind of impression you are making on so many, many people you pass casually in your life. It could be the checkout girl at Walmart that you compliment on her blue eyes or the sad grocery store teenager that carries out your groceries. Life here on earth is not easy for anyone. Every person you meet has loved something, is afraid of something, and has lost something. And as Pierre Teilhard de Chardin said so beautifully, "We are not human beings having a spiritual experience. We are spiritual beings having a human experience."

To truly have self-confidence and to make a good lasting impression, you must first know yourself (the reason for this book) and then discover God's purpose for you (the reason for your life). When you dress in the morning using the techniques you have now learned, do not forget to put on God's armor for the day as well. He offers us the gifts of love, joy, peace, patience, kindness, goodness, faithfulness, gentleness, and self-control. When you are armed with His strength for living, He will give you true confidence. This confidence comes from knowing God created you as a special, unique being. You have a future that no one else on this earth was created to live.

And just as I remembered my first-grade student's name so well, God knows your name so well too. You are special to Him, and this thought is more important than how you dress. I truly believe that using our time and money wisely glorifies God. If I didn't believe that, I wouldn't have spent so much time writing this book just for you. But even more than that truth is the truth of your uniqueness and the wonderful piece you are in God's puzzle we call life. Without you, the puzzle wouldn't be complete!

So to finish this book, I want to tell all of my readers, customers through the years, students I have taught in so many capacities, friends I love so dearly, and family I am truly blessed with that I love you—but even more importantly, *God loves you!*

So dress for *His* success, dear woman of God, give *Him* the glory, and your true beauty will never fade.

Notes

Epilogue

"What is Beautiful"

What is Love? What is Truth and Kindness?
Why is the *Mona Lisa* a work of Beauty?
Describe the fragrance of the Blue Iris. . . .

Is Beauty not a Gestalt, beyond definition?
One knows Beauty when present.
It involves all of our senses,
Is felt, seen, smelled, tasted, and heard. . . .

Might I propose in our perfectly imperfect world,
We encounter glimpses of Beauty.
Providing Hope and Perseverance,
And a knowledge of something more. . . .

Might I propose Absolute Beauty is the Divine.
When that day arrives, Beauty upon beauty. . . .
You kneel and He asks you to stand.
You're prompted for one statement. . . .

And your reply is "Thank You."

—Scott Tallent

Notes

Notes

Notes

Notes

For more information about
TICA TALLENT
&
WHAT IS BEAUTIFUL:
SECRETS FROM A PERSONAL SHOPPER
please visit:

www.ticatallent.com
tica@ticatallent.com

· ·

For more information about
AMBASSADOR INTERNATIONAL
please visit:

www.ambassador-international.com
@AmbassadorIntl
www.facebook.com/AmbassadorIntl

Warm Colors

OLIVE GREEN

LIGHT GRAY

YELLOW GREEN

TURQUOISE

CAMEL

ORANGE

IVORY

CORAL

PEACH

APRICOT

GOLD

BROWN

PERIWINKLE

LIGHT RED

Cool Colors

PINK

ORCHID

HOT PINK

FUCHSIA

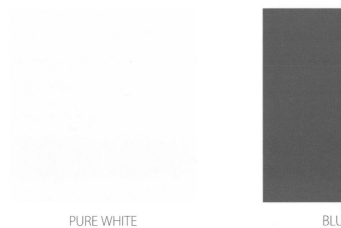

PURE WHITE

BLUE GREEN

MEDIUM BLUE

BLUE GRAY

LAVENDER

PURPLE

DARK BLUE

PLUM

DARK RED

BURGUNDY

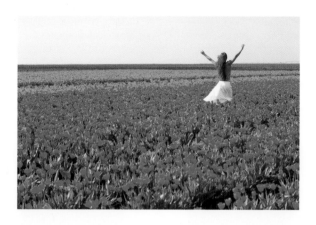

*"Finally, brethren, whatever is true, whatever
is honorable, whatever is right, whatever is
pure, whatever is lovely, whatever is of good
repute, if there is any excellence and if anything
worthy of praise, dwell on these things."*

—Philippians 4:8